# Contents

# Introduction

I'm sure you have been realized that obesity is an epidemic that affects all the persons and all age groups. This problem assumes an alarming situation in Western nations due to abundant food available here.

## Is Obesity an eternal problem?

If you can understand the psyche of obese people that losing weight is insurmountable problem. On the face of this statement you may disagree with

me. However, the way the weight loss industry is growing and number of weight loss diets coming up on regular intervals validates my statement beyond any doubt.

## Perception problem

Listen up! Unless you change this wrong perception and come to the reality, the obesity problem continuously haunts you without any hope of becoming lean and healthy.

## Eat less

Remember! The simple truth is that you have piled up excess fat by eating excess calories than what is required for your body. The obvious solution is that you have to prepare a diet with fewer calories so your calorie intake will come down.

## It is not that simple

That seems to be very easier to say than do. Okay I can understand but the fact remains that in order to lose weight, intake of calories must be less than your body required and that is how your excess fat will be burned.

## The solution is in your hands

Despite of this simple fact, there is Sea of misinformation available all over the Internet and other mediums that are complicating instead of solving the problem. As a consequence, the obesity rates are growing in alarming proportions. Today an average American body fat has become higher with disastrous health consequences.

Okay let's see what the consequences of excess body fat are:

- It is an undeniable fact that carrying an excess fat will have impact on physical and emotional life.

- It has been estimated that obesity related conditions cost of over 150 million dollars and cause 300,000 premature deaths in US alone.

- High blood pressure, diabetes, heart diseases, joint problems, cancer, and many psychological disorders are said to be associated with obesity.

**bodyweight training**

It's so simple… but bodyweight training might well be the one thing you need to start making some major changes in your life.

Not to say that you necessarily *need* to be making changes… But if you're looking for a way to build more muscle, to lose fat, to feel healthier and better about yourself and to be pumped full of energy – bodyweight training can do all that.

And this is true *even if* you have failed to get into shape with other training programs in the past. In fact, bodyweight training is the perfect antidote for anyone who has struggled with regular workouts. Whether you tried running, lifting weights or anything else – bodyweight training presents an answer that is easier, faster and more effective – and that's more likely to help you get the results you're looking for.

Even if you *have* been successful with other programs in the past – bodyweight training can be the perfect addition to your routine and can help you to get even better benefits even more quickly. And it's a different *kind* of fitness and strength you'll enjoy too. You'll be strong but you'll also be perfectly proportioned, more full of energy and even more agile.

Bodyweight training gives you power like a coiled spring!

At this point, the first question you might be asking is: why bodyweight training? What's so different about working out with your own body? Why do people succeed with this type of exercise when all else has failed? Let's take a look at some pretty convincing reasons that bodyweight training is what you need…

## The Many Benefits of Bodyweight Training

**#1 Practical Benefits**

For starters, bodyweight training has a ton of practical benefits that a lot of other types of exercise just can't deliver.

For starters, bodyweight training doesn't require *any* equipment or tools. As we'll see later on, there are some items that can help you to get more from your training and a pull up bar in particular is highly advisable. Nevertheless though, this still isn't a *requirement* by any stretch and you can get away without one. Even if you do go for a pull up bar, this is something that can fit into your doorframe and that won't set you back more than $5 at a push.

This right away is something that gives bodyweight training a big advantage. This means that you don't have to spend any cash to get started with it and it means that you can do it anywhere. A lot of people like to use bodyweight training when visiting hotels and other places they can stay and you can even do this kind of training when you're camping!

But this also makes it much easier to get started in your own home. The fact of the matter is that many of us can't afford to invest in expensive gym equipment like bench presses or squat racks and most of us don't have the room anyway!

Then there's the fact that having lots of equipment means it's actually quite a lot of work in order to start training. If you're going to be using dumbbells, barbells, a bench, a kettlebell… this means that you're going to have get all of that equipment out and set it up to use. That might not sound like a big deal but if you live in a small space it can involve quite a lot of work and it can add 10 minutes to you training. Bearing in mind that you need to pack it away again, this can be the difference between a quick, spontaneous workout or not having time to train at all.

With bodyweight training, there's nothing stopping you from getting a quick 5 minute workout in even when you're waiting at the bus stop. And as we'll see, this is a really great way to train as it means you're no longer spending most of your day sedentary and going all-out for just one hour. Using bodyweight training we can be much more tactical and versatile in the way we train and *when* we train.

**#2 Physical Benefits**

Another thing to consider is the way that bodyweight training can impact on your body. Of course any type of exercise should help you to get fitter, stronger and leaner… that's rather the point!

But what bodyweight does better than any other type of exercise is to help you build a powerful 'strength to weight ratio'. This basically means that you can become *very* strong without gaining a lot of extra weight.

At the same time, bodyweight training is very active. The very nature of it means that you're using your whole body when you do that kind of training and that means that your heartrate goes up, you burn more fat and you improve your energy levels.

When you workout at the gym, a lot of the exercise you'll do actually involves lying down! You'll lie down while you perform the bench press for instance and you'll sit down while doing bicep curls a lot of the time. This will get your heartrate up to around 80 – maybe – but press ups are far more active and can get it up to 110 and above.

Better yet, bodyweight training teaches you how to use your whole body to become more agile and quick. Bodyweight training often includes elements of balance, of flexibility and of explosive power – and all these things contribute to improved health and performance across the board.

If you want to be fast, lean, light and powerful – then nothing quite beats bodyweight training.

**#3 It's Fun!**

Believe it or not, bodyweight training can be a lot of fun. We've already seen that it's much easier, more practical and more active than weights training. But at the same time, you'll find that bodyweight training helps you to learn cool party tricks, skills and abilities that make it so much more worthwhile. If you get really good for instance, then you can start to pull of feats of strength like one-armed pull ups, clapping press-ups and even handstand press ups. This is incredibly rewarding and gives you an awesome sense of progression.

Bodyweight training is also a lot more versatile than other types of training and it lets you work out in different ways that almost feel like games. You can do bodyweight training outdoors, or you can do it using some kind of ball or other tool to turn it into a sport.

What You Will Learn

As you can see then, bodyweight training has a *ton* of advantages: it's easy, fun, practical, quick, versatile and it's very effective and good for you.

There's a problem though and that's that a lot of people just don't know how to make bodyweight training work for them.

## 1. Flexible

Unlike other diets, the fast diet is easy to stick on for a long term that is why this really works. You eat normally for five days and reduce your calories only for two days a week. So this flexibility is not available in other diets as you have to reduce your calories every day.

Another important benefit of this diet is that this lifestyle will not come into your way as you can attend parties and go to business lunches....

## 2. Enjoyable

Once you realize that there are five days in a week in which you can eat anything you want, you can enjoy the fast diet lifestyle.

You can do a fasting twice in nonconsecutive days during Monday to Friday, which are the days you are generally busy. As you are preoccupied with work the sign of hunger doesn't affect you much. As a whole you love this lifestyle.

## 3. No need to avoid your favorite foods

Unlike other popular diets the fast diet lifestyle does not suggest you to eliminate your favorite foods for weight loss.

Those who are on fast diet eat normally for five days a week. This is what we call as a feed time. During feeding time you can eat whatever the food you like normal and there is no restriction whatsoever.

The only thing you have to keep in mind is that don't over stuff during this time to ensure that the benefits that you derive during fasting time are maintained.

## 4. No restrictions

The problem with many other diets is that you have to follow a super restrictive diet for a long period of time. Only a small set of people who are very dedicated can follow this strict regiment and achieve phenomenal results. However, for many people following such strict regiment's practically impossible. Even though they follow for certain period of time, they give up in the middle and as a result the weight loss process comes to a grinding halt.

Unlike other types the fast diet doesn't require to follow restrictive dietary regiment. In fact this diet not interferes with your regular lifestyle, so you can lose weight steadily while eating your favorite foods.

## 5. Can be followed easily

After following the fast diet for a couple of months, I'm sure you will feel that you have found an eating plan that you will be following for life time. You don't experience this feeling in the other diets.

## 6. Permanent results

I understand that the goal of any weight loss program is a permanent weight loss. Nobody wants a program that is short lived.

But it is a fact that many weight loss programs that promises quick weight loss finally end up with weight gain. And this is the main reason that people switchover to different weight loss programs with the hope of permanent results.

Remember that any diet that is not flexible enough and also too much restrictive doesn't bring permanent results.

Thankfully is the fast diet lifestyle being very flexible and not restrictive in the sense that you will not feel deprived of your food choices, the result of your weight loss is permanent.

You have to realize that the fasting is a method of weight loss that can only bring last longing results.

## 7. It is a lifestyle

If I say that fast diet is a diet program, I am simply looking at its surface rather than going deep inside of it. I therefore urge upon you not to consider this as a diet program rather than a lifestyle.

By embracing this attitude you can quickly adopt a fast diet as your lifestyle and fully enjoy all the health benefits associated with it.

Factually, fast diet is a lifestyle because it does not stipulate any timing, recommend any foods, and impose restrictions on your favorite diets.

## 8. No side-effects

Most of the fad diets not healthy and eventually leaves you with many side effects such as fatigue, nausea and other disorders

It is also reported that over the counter HCG products that are used for weight loss are not good for your health.

There are a lot of risks associated with rapid weight loss which includes malnutrition, dehydration and electrolyte imbalances.

The fast diet lifestyle does not entail any extreme forms of intervention into your body functioning and therefore it will not have any side effects.

## 9. It doesn't take your time and energy

With the fast diet lifestyle you can live an active and healthy life without taking your time and energy. This is possible due to the fact that there is no need of searching for more diets.

The main benefit of fast diet lifestyle is that you can eat the foods that you like. You don't try to classify which foods are good and which foods are bad. You are in full charge of your food regiment and therefore you enjoy peace of mind.

## 10. Inexpensive

Fast diet lifestyle does not recommend any expensive supplements or foods. It is simply restricting the calorie intake for a 24-hour period twice in a week. And that's it.

Weight loss is a balancing act of feeding and fasting

Your body is designed to eat, store and burn.

That means we're always live in two states i.e feeding and fasting.

In the feeding state we eat and store the food. In the fasting state we burn the food.

In other words your body is designed to eat the food and store in the form of fat when it is available. When the food is scarce, your body uses food that is stored in fats.

Your body is not yet upgraded:

What do I mean by "not upgraded body" it means that your body is designed and functions to tune with ancient conditions, when food is not available 24 x 7.

In olden days your ancestors hunt for food and there is no guarantee of availability always. In those conditions you have to necessarily store the food to meet the contingencies.

## Food abundance

Fortunately today there is no shortage of food for the people like us living in Western nations. That means there is no need for us to excessively eat and store in the form of fats. However the reality is that we eat in excess quantities, unable to resist the temptations of tasty colorful foods that are marketed by food industry. The resultant condition is that we are a nation of obese people facing many problems.

## Fasting is the only way out to lose weight:

Fasting is the only way to maintain the calorie balance. Put it simply store some fat when you are eating and burn some fat when you're not eating.

## You fast everyday

Remember! Fasting is not a new phenomenon. You are fasting everyday when you are sleeping. If you sleep for eight hours obviously you are fasting for eight hours. In order to lose weight you have to extend the period of fasting to some more extra hours. And that's it.

## Conscious fasting

Now the question is that when your body is designed for feeding and also fasting why not people consciously take up fasting for weight loss?

## Age-old practice

You may not aware that in the Eastern societies the habit of fasting has been impregnated into their culture and therefore fasting is part of their daily routine.

In Western societies, the concept of fasting has been disappeared in the wake of consumerism and therefore the concept of fasting appears to be Greek and Latin.

replace your existing food habits with new ones. That is to say that the fast diet lifestyle can help you unlearn your past food habits and replace them with healthy ones.

So when you shifted to fast diet lifestyle you may experience some sort of dizziness initially and however as you move through it all such tendencies will disappear.

**Myth#5: fasting will make you lightheaded**

It is a fact that low sugars in your blood can cause lightheadedness. We call this state as hypoglycemic. This is a common symptom for those who are suffering with diabetes.

**Fast diet is not a full fast**

If you go for full 24 hours fast even then you will not have any problem of hypoglycemic state. Obviously since the fast diet lifestyle that I am talking now is not a full fast and as it is semi-fast the symptoms of dizziness is almost ruled out.

**Anxiety and stress related**

Despite of all these facts if you experience the symptoms of lightheadedness when you are on fast diet, this may be caused by anxiety and stress.

**Apprehensions about fasting**

People have many apprehensions about fasting. This includes a wrong belief system of fasting is unhealthy. In some cases these symptoms may be caused by the very feeling of not eating the food that they like. This we call as royal symptoms.

**Fast diet is for healthy people**

So fasting is not advisable for those who suffer with diabetes. In healthy individuals fasting does not cause low blood sugars. Initial symptoms of lightheadedness will be subsided in the course of time. In view of these facts you should not give up your fast diet lifestyle simply based on your apprehensions.

## Fast diet is a lifestyle

Let me emphasize that the fast diet is not a diet program. Here I am not suggesting any weight loss foods or any weight loss meal plans.

The fast diet is a simple strategy of reducing intake of calories to optimally maintain bodyweight and burning excess fat. It is a holistic and healthy lifestyle with any health benefits associated with it.

### Focus on calories but not on food

In the fast diet lifestyle the focus is reducing the calorie intake but not on foods that we eat. It is aimed at reducing the quantity of food that we eat every day. It is estimated that on an average most of the Americans are eating almost 4000 cal of food each day and that is double what we typically need in a day.

### 24-hour mini fasts

So it is a way of life where you embrace the idea of taking 24 hour mini fasts twice in a week so as to reduce overall intake of food.

### Fast diet for weight loss

You have to realize that the simplest way to lose weight, maintain your lean muscle and enjoy all the health benefits is by giving rest to your body couple of times in a week. Importantly it is the only way you can get rid of your compulsive eating habits
Fast diet is easy

The fast diet lifestyle is not only easy but also inexpensive as it doesn't require expensive foods and supplements. The only thing you have to do is restrict the quantity of food you take at least two days a week.

### intermittent mini fasting

Even though the fast diet food habits are ancient and it is common in most Eastern traditions, the British physician Dr Michael Mosley propagated this strategy first in England then be displayed to other nations.

As I told you elsewhere the fast diet is not a diet plan. It is change of a lifestyle to achieve a permanent weight loss along with many other health benefits.

**Feeding five days & fasting two days**

The fast diet is also called as 5:2 intermittent fasting diet. This simply means you eat the food in regular way for five days a week. On two days during the week you reduce the intake of calories down to a total of 600 cal in case of men and 500 cal in case of women. In any given point of time the fasting period must not be more than 24 hours.

500 or 600 cal is not a lot and yet it is enough to function and workout without any difficulty.

**Don't extend fasting periods**

Remember! You don't extend fasting periods of time in your anxiety to lose weight fast. This is because extended period of fasting is turning your body into a starvation mode thereby slowing down its metabolism.

**How the fast diet burn excess fat?**

When you are on fasting diet, the body looks for the stored food in the body to meet its energy requirements and that is how your body functions properly. After taking all the glucose in your blood, it turns into the glycogen that is stored in your liver and muscle tissues. Once the glycogen is used, the body will start burning the fat for its energy and that is how you lose your excess fat.

**Preferred foods?**

You can include lean protein sources and lots of vegetables for your fasting day menu. You're not mindful of low calorie intake as this meal seems to be more substantial.

Just wait till tomorrow!

When you start you feel it hard but not terrible as such. However, as you continue with this lifestyle you feel better. And when you feel hunger, just remember, that you have to wait until tomorrow. If you still cannot resist the hungry you can have an amazing cup of green tea and your hunger goes away.

**Fast days**

During fast days you may eat one meal in the evening and tried to keep it around 500 or 600 calories limit. If you wish to spread it twice you can do so by following calories limit.

**Feeding days**

On your feed days you can eat pretty much normally but don't overdo it... but you still can eat sweets, burgers, and chips.

**Workout during fast diet lifestyle**

Many people who are on fast diet have a doubt that whether they can continue to work out during fasting. There is no need to stop your workout when you fast. And one more thing if you continue your workout even during fast time you will notice improved stamina.

**Fast diet + workouts**

Combining your fast diet lifestyle with some kind of workout preferably with weights is desirable to maintain the muscle mass.

A regular workout along with your fast diet lifestyle will have number of benefits. Besides maintaining and building your muscle during fasting, it also affects your self esteem and your body image. As a whole you not only lose your weight but also feel good about yourself.

## *Fasting in religions*

### Fasting in Christianity

The purpose of fasting is to focus on prayer. Some Christians skip couple of meals a day. Some Christians abstain from food full day or even longer periods of time.

### Fasting and praying go together

Christians believe that fasting is a means to establish a Rapport with the God. They also believe that fasting has to be done privately with absolute immunity otherwise they will not derive any benefits out of it. As a whole fasting and prayer will go hand-in-hand in the Christian life.

## Fasting in Islam

We all know that Muslims spent a whole month fasting and prayers. They follow total abstinence from food and drink from dawn to dusk.

## The spirit of virtue

The main purpose of fasting and praying is to inculcate the spirit of virtue. That is why they don't take anything from morning to evening in the month of Ramadan.

## Fasting in Hinduism

Hindus believe that it is not practically possible to live a life of spirituality in their daily life. It is true that we are distracted by many indulgences that do not allow us to lead a spiritual life.

## Hindus practice the fast diet

In general Hindus fast certain days in a week depending on their choice of God or Goddess. It is also a common practice that during festival time they fast.

## Fasting will detox

Ayurveda is ancient Indian medical system wherein the underlying principles of fasting were clearly mentioned. As per ayurveda system all the diseases are caused by accumulation of toxic material in the digestive system. By giving rest to the digestive system it can cleanse and correct the imbalance in the body naturally.

## Fasting our way of life

If you can deeply understand the cultural practices of all the religions, you can realize the importance of fasting in our lives. So the fast diet lifestyle that is being propagated today is in fact not a new diet. Fast diet lifestyle is meant to help people maintaining health and lead a peaceful life.

### Benefits of fast diet lifestyle

Intermittent fasting is the most effective and easy way to cut the calories; lose excess body fat and also gives amazing health benefits.

**It really works for your weight loss**

If you follow the fast diet method you can see weight loss in 4 to 6 weeks time. It is also best to keep your weight under control for a long time. The best thing is that even you eat a dessert you will not feel any guilty because the fast diet lifestyle has been designed on the premise of that you should not be deprived of your fabric foods.

**You feel more energetic**

The fast diet lifestyle is relatively easy to follow and it doesn't feel you are on a diet. Gradually your blood count will improve and as such you feel more energetic and lively.

**Lose obsession with food**

The difficult thing for anyone who wants to go on a diet is a lot of misinformation about fasting.

And that is why they post pone fasting always. Now, as you know the concept of intermittent fasting you no longer dislike fasting because you know that you can eat tomorrow anything you like. In view of this eventually you lose your obsession with food.

**Fast diet lowers glucose levels**

Apart from losing excess pounds it can also lowers your blood glucose levels. This helps to diabetic patients also.

**Naturally increase growth hormone**

Growth hormone helps burning the fat, building the muscle and also has anti-ageing effect. It is also responsible for maintaining your lean body mass. Over weight and abdominal fat can suppress the secretion of growth hormone.

There are three ways to increase growth hormones in your body. I.e Fasting, exercise and relaxed sleeping.

**Celebrities pay but you don't**

The good news is that fasting can cause large increase of growth hormone in all age groups. That means you can have natural growth hormone by simply fasting which otherwise the celebrities are paying thousands of dollars.

**Improvement of overall health and life span**

Prolonged and chronic inflammation is one of the key factors for life-threatening diseases including rheumatoid arthritis, hypertension, fatty liver, cardio vascular diseases and diabetes.

**Fasting keeps inflammation under control**

Chronic inflammation is widespread in people with obesity. Intermittent fasting combined with regular workouts will help you to get rid of excess fat. Excess fat and over eating are main causes of inflammation.

Fast diet lifestyle automatically keeps inflammation under control and thereby improves your health and longevity.

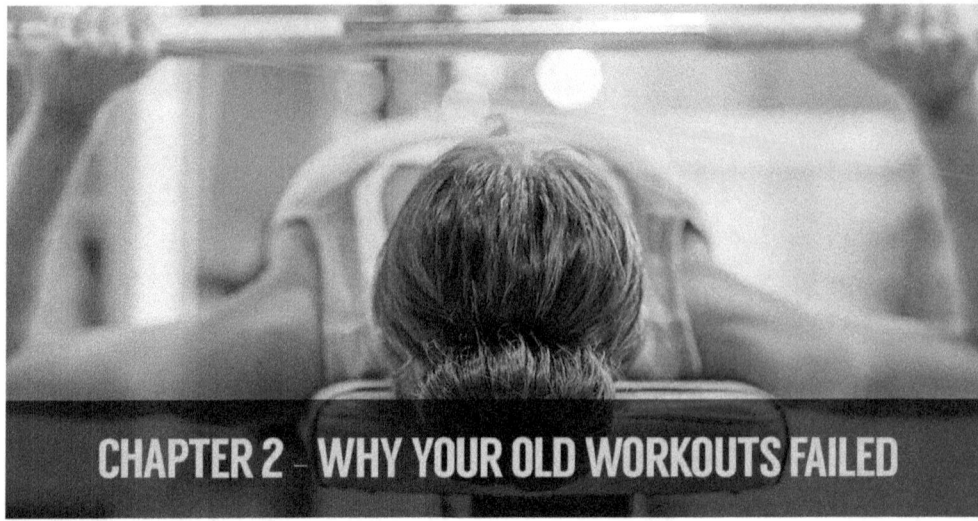

**CHAPTER 2 – WHY YOUR OLD WORKOUTS FAILED**

## Chapter 2. Why Your Old Workouts Failed

Think about how many people you know who have tried to get into shape and failed. Think about how many of your friends or family members have started new training programs or new weight loss regimes. Either they're trying to build big muscle, or they're interested in losing fat.

Either way, they come to you all excited about their new goals and they show you their program. Often it will involve training five days a week at the gym, perhaps for an hour at a time.

At the same time, this new training program is going to involve eating 500 fewer calories.

How can it possibly fail?

I'll tell you how it fails. In fact, I'll tell you how it fails nearly *every single time*.

The problem isn't that the training program isn't good. The problem is that they don't stick at it.

They have this exciting aim and they're all ready to get going with it, but by week two they're already losing motivation.

Something 'important' comes up and they have to take a day out of training. Either that or they just get home from work and they're so tired they have to skip a session…

Then they get a cold and that means another week off.

And their friends are eating out and they're invited, so they head to that and they consume

1,500 calories in one sitting. So far, so bad.

By the end of week three, they're now back at the position they were in *to begin with* and they've made no progress on their diet or their training. This is disheartening and it's also somewhat *embarrassing* when people ask them how their fitness is going.

So they just kind of brush it to one side and then pretend that it never happened. Until the next program comes along that is!

You're probably very familiar with this story and in fact, it's probably a story that you've *lived* yourself a lot of times.

The problem is that these training programs are just too ambitious. Taking on a new training program like this takes an *incredible* amount of dedication and energy.

Think about it: right now you probably feel like you don't have much time in your life. You probably feel rushed off your feet and you probably have very little energy when you get back in the evenings.

*This* is why you're currently out of shape. It's not for lack of interest or for lack of trying. If it were easy to get into incredible shape, then you would have done it already! Truth is that life is hard and most of us are struggling just to keep afloat.

Here's a quick newsflash by the way: time isn't the problem.

All of us think that we have a problem with time but this is almost always untrue. We very often think that we don't have time and that's why we don't get everything we want done. But if that's true, then how come you were able to watch that entire boxset of Game of Thrones recently? How come you spent all of last night just lying in front of the TV?

How come you were able to hit snooze three times on your alarm?

The problem isn't time – it's energy. Energy is finite and there's only so much stress and so much work/activity that we can cram into one day before that finite energy begins to run dry.

If you're *already* at your wits end. If you're already exhausted and stressed… then wh makes you think that you can add a workout to the end of your day that's an hour long And what makes you think that you can drive *to* the gym to do your workout? And the back? And then shower?

There are more things about going to the gym that we don't take into account too. F instance, the cost. Then there's the cold weather.

And here's one: all that extra washing! If you go to the gym 5 days a week, then you be creating five more pairs of dirty underwear and you'll need to wash all those joggir bottoms and tank tops…

You expect to do all this when you *already* have no energy and you also intend to e fewer calories? Giving yourself *even less* energy?

And you wonder why so many training programs fail?

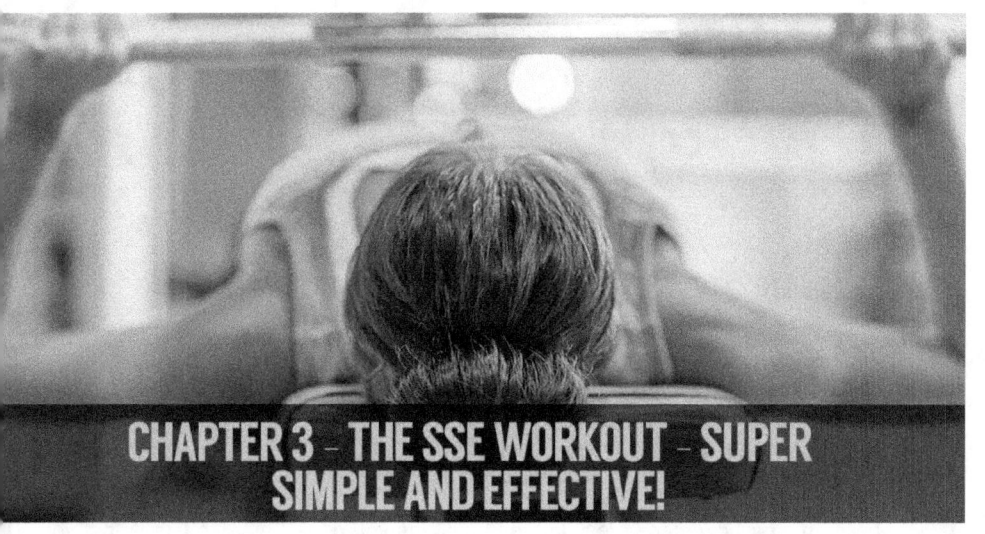

CHAPTER 3 - THE SSE WORKOUT - SUPER SIMPLE AND EFFECTIVE!

## Chapter 3. The SSE Workout – Super Simple and Effective!

I want to demonstrate the power of bodyweight training to you right away and that's why I'm starting with this simple workout. It's called the 'SSE' workout because it's super simple and effective.

This is a workout that addresses *all* of the issues that we saw in the last chapter and then some.

It's a workout that takes 10-15 minutes. All you need is a pull up bar (or a tree branch). And you're going to do it in the morning, before you shower.

### The Workout

The workout is a circuit. That means that you'll go through each exercise once and then you're going to start again from the beginning.

You're going to rest for 30 seconds between each completed set and you're going to perform each set of moves for 30 seconds.

The exercises are push ups, pull ups and jack in the box.

So the workout looks like this:

- ☐ 30 seconds of push ups

- ☐ 30 seconds of pull ups

- ☐ 30 seconds of jack in the box

- ☐ 30 seconds of rest

You then repeat it five times.

Make sure that you are doing as many repetitions of each exercise as you can and that you're giving it your all. You also need to ensure that you aren't resting *at all* when you move from one to the next.

It doesn't matter how many press ups and pull ups you do. All that matters is that you keep going until the end of the thirty seconds (at least keep trying).

If you can't do push ups, then you can do push ups on your knees to begin with.

And if you can't do pull ups (or can't do enough), then you're going to do *assisted* pull ups.

Assisted pull ups means that you're going to take a chair and put it underneath the pull up bar.

You can now put your feet on that chair and use them to slightly help yourself through each pull up. Don't cheat and just 'stand up' – just give yourself the slightest bit of help with your legs so that you can complete each exercise.

Remember as well that pull ups are the ones where you use an overhand (pronated) grip. That means that your palms are facing away from you and this way, you'll also be engaging your lats more in the exercise rather than your biceps.

Finally, when performing the jack-in-the-box, you need to squat all the way down and crouch, then you're exploding upward and splaying your arms and legs like a star-fish. It's like a squat combined with a star jump. If you can't do this, then just tuck jumps will be fine to begin with.

That's the whole workout. Like I said, it's simple. But it's also really effective.

And you're going to do it five days a week before you start work.

One more tip: don't do it immediately upon waking. Wait at least 10 minutes as that way your spine won't be soft from sleeping and you'll reduce the chances of injury. This is pretty light stuff though, so you should find you're fine to go into it without a warm up.

## Why This Works

So what's so special about this workout?

The first thing is that it has everything you need in it. The workout has three components: push, pull and legs. Each exercise is also compound and that way, you're actually targeting *nearly* every muscle in the body:

**Press ups**: Pecs, triceps, shoulders, traps, abs

**Pull ups**: Lats, biceps, abs

**Jack in the Box**: Quads, hamstrings, calves, glutes

You're also going fast and all of these exercises are enough to get your heart rating. That means that if you go as intense as you can, you can easily stand to burn around 150 calories from this alone. At the start of your day that's an *excellent* way to begin and it means you can slip up and eat a KitKat without it mattering as much. By the way, that also adds up to 750 calories by the end of the week...

And because you're training at the start of the day – before breakfast – this counts as 'fasted cardio'. For those who don't know, this basically means you're performing cardiovascular exercise at a point where there is no glucose in your blood. That in turn means that the body will burn *fat* rather than sugar and you'll lose more weight as a result.

Then there's the fact that these moves are actually *quite* tough in terms of the muscle work. You can easily start to notice your biceps, your pecs and your abs strengthen from this alone. Press ups are actually *surprisingly* good for your abs. Not only because you're training fast enough to burn calories but because you'll be using your transverse abdominis (the abdominal muscle that wraps around your body like a weight belt) in order to hold your stomach in. This will make your abs look much flatter and it's what's missing from a lot of training programs.

Better yet, this is also *super* convenient. No matter how much of a rush you're in or how tired you are, almost everyone can afford to get up 10 minutes earlier and do 10 minutes of exercise. You need to be strict with yourself here: never go over the 10 minutes. This defies the object and means you'll end up putting it off.

You're doing *just* 10 minutes. But it's enough to build more strength, more energy and more lean muscle mass.

The other big advantage is that you're doing this before your shower. And you can wear the clothes you slept in! Just some underwear will be fine even because you're training in the comfort of your own home. So in a pair of boxer shorts or panties, you can perform your press ups and pulls and then jump straight in the shower.

Now you aren't having an 'extra' shower that takes up time and you don't have any more clothes to wash. This is a ten-minute workout that *really is* only ten minutes long!

This is something that *everyone* can afford to add to their regime therefore and it's enough to help you lose more weight, build more muscle and generally get a lot stronger and fitter.

If you already workout regularly – even if you're an athlete or a bodybuilder – then just adding this little bit of extra training at the start of your day will be enough to help you through patches where you miss workouts and to ensure you get that little bit more exercise throughout the day. Simply put, the SSE workout is the solution to all of your training problems

– so add it to your regime!

Now you have something to start doing right away… so start doing it!

Don't wait until you've read the rest of this book. Don't wait until you've spoken with a personal trainer.

All that really matters, is that you start doing *something*. You'll learn more as we go through the book but in the meantime just start doing that one thing and start making progress!

*Variations*

As you get a little more advanced, you might start to find that the 'SSE' workout is a little *too* simplistic. Or maybe you want to adapt it to be a little more 'total body'.

In that case, you can do so by simply adding some extra moves to your regime and swapping them in and out:

- [ ] Dips (you can do this with two chairs opposite one another)

- [ ] Tricep dips

- [ ] Chin ups

- [ ] Incline press ups

st make sure that you have one compound push movement, one pull and one ercise for the legs!

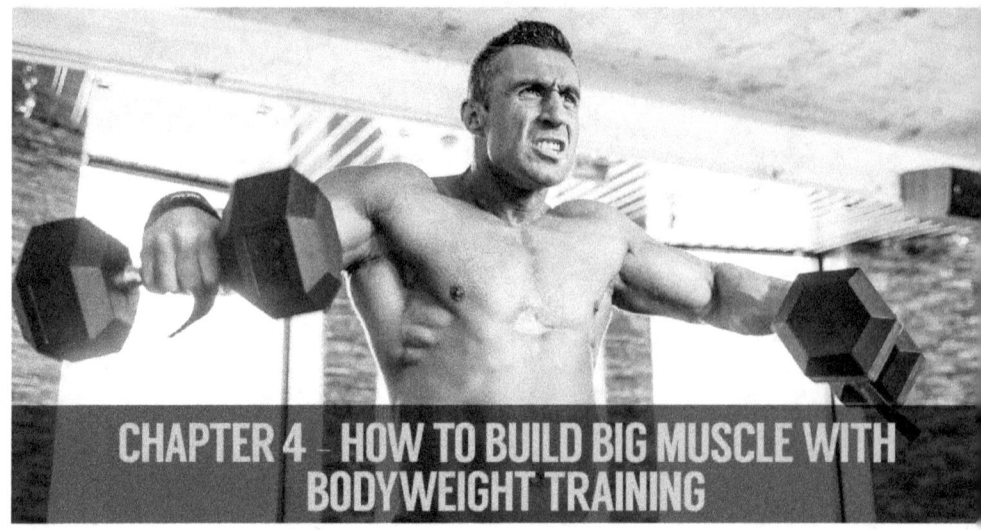

## Chapter 4. How to Build BIG Muscle With Bodyweight Training

Using the SSE workout, you can start getting fitter and burning fat/building muscle right away.

But what if you want to become the next Arnold Schwarzenegger? What if you want to become incredibly bulky, ripped and hench? In that case, you might think that your only option is to start lifting weights but you would be wrong – in fact there are a number of ways you can build big muscle using bodyweight alone and it's probably a lot easier than you suspect.

In this chapter, we're going to be looking at how building muscle works and we're going to look at how you can do it using bodyweight. This is all about theory. Towards the end of the book we'll be looking at the individual bodyweight moves you can use and providing a kind of glossary of exercises for you to dip in and out of. So read this and then apply it to those moves. Although to be honest, you can do most of this with just the regular few bodyweight exercises you probably already know.

So let's take a look at how to build muscle…

### The Science of Hypertrophy

Muscle growth in response to training is technically known as 'hypertrophy'. Hypertrophy is what bodybuilding is all about and if you're trying to look big and bulky, it's what you need to be all about as well.

So the question is: how does hypertrophy work? How can you stimulate your body to produce more muscle?

And the answer is that you need to provide the body with *volume*. Volume is what defines the intensity of your training and it can come either from increasing the weight or from increasing the number of repetitions. Or both.

This then triggers changes in the muscle that causes it to grow and there is widely believed to be two different mechanisms through which this can occur:

- Sarcoplasmic hypertrophy

- Myofibrillar hypertrophy

## Sarcoplasmic Hypertrophy

Sarcoplasmic hypertrophy is the type of hypertrophy that is caused when you increase the number of repetitions. This is the kind of muscle growth that you get when you train with rep-ranges of around 12-15 or even higher. It's also increased when you increase your 'time under tension' which is the amount of time you spend actually straining under the weight (rather than setting it down to rest between sets).

When you increase the number of repetitions you perform and when you hold the weight in position, you are calling on your muscle's endurance. This in turn relies on the amount of fluid and the amount of energy (ATP) stored in the muscle cells – the sarcoplasm.

When you use this kind of training, it means that the muscle is constantly tensed and working.

In turn, this causes the blood to 'occlude'. In other words, it gets sent to the muscle and it stays there. This is also what causes us to get the feeling of 'pump' when we're working out. As this happens, you also get a build-up of metabolites – muscle-building products that are found in the blood and that end up flooding the muscles. Metabolites include the likes of testosterone, growth hormone and IGF1. You also get a lot of nutrients in here.

As a result, the muscle responds by growing and specifically by swelling and taking on more water mass. This gives the muscles a bigger, bloated look. They may be quite 'soft' but it's a great way to get big fast and to increase your ability to perform large sets of exercise.

## Sarcoplasmic Hypertrophy

Another thing that occurs as you train is that you create tiny tears in the muscle fiber. These are called 'microtears' and they're so small as to not be damaging in any way or that painful (although this can lead to 'DOMS' the next day – delayed onset muscle soreness).

What these microtears *can* do though, is to cause the muscle to appear damaged to the body and that means it needs to get repaired. When you're resting later on then, the body will use protein from your diet in order to rebuild the muscle and each of those muscle fibers will come back slightly thicker and slightly stronger than before. This increases size *and* strength and the best way to trigger this kind of hypertrophy is by training with heavy weights. This is how

'power lifters' will train and it's how they manage to get very strong lifting a weight only a few times.

What you also need to know about is the different types of muscle fiber. Your muscles have a number of different 'kinds' of muscle fibers that make them up and each has a slightly different role. In general though, we can split these muscle fibers into two categories which are 'fast twitch' and 'slow twitch'. Fast twitch fibers are capable of creating greater acceleration and greater force – and that means that they are the most useful kinds for lifting heavy weights. Your body will use these first when you move heavy weight and once they've become fatigued/torn, it will move on to the slower twitch fibers. Eventually, you don't have enough power to move the weight – but some slow twitch fibers will remain which will mean you're still able to move your arms!

## *Building Strength*

There's something else that occurs here too though and that's that you are also strengthening your 'mind muscle connection'. This is the ability of your brain to actually *use* the muscle you've got in order to exert force and the more you train, the greater that ability becomes.

Each time you contract a muscle, you do so by sending signals from your brain through your central nervous system. When that signal reaches the end of the nerve, acetylcholine is released across the 'neuromuscular junction' and this causes the muscle cells to fire.

As you do this repeatedly, you are actually able to increase the number of nuclei in your muscle cells (called myonuclei) which means that more of your muscle fibers can fire in response to that signal. This *also* contributes to extra muscle growth, because the number of nuclei is directly related to protein synthesis – the ability of the muscles to use the protein in your diet to build muscle!

## Making Sense of the Science

That's a lot of science to take on board but don't worry if you don't follow it all.

All you really need to know is that lifting weights creates tears in the muscle fiber and builds up the amount of fluids in the muscle cells and that both these processes contribute to muscle growth and strength increases.

Both these processes also hurt slightly. No matter what anyone tells you (and some people try to deny this), working out to build muscle *should* be uncomfortable.

It's a very specific type of pain and you shouldn't push it too far. But building up lactic acid

(which accumulates along with the metabolites) and tearing the muscle both cause the muscle to burn during your training and the next day. Ask any bodybuilder or athlete and they'll say the same thing. 'No pain, no gain'.

Now the trouble we face is going to be trying to get the muscle to grow using only our own bodyweight.

If you're training with weights this is easy. All you have to do is add an extra 10kg to your bar and you've made it more difficult.

But if you're training with your body, then things get significantly harder. Once you can do 100 press ups, how can you make it more difficult?
Fortunately, there are a number of tricks and methods we can use…

The good news is that your body doesn't *care* whether you're lifting a heavy weight or not. As far as your body is concerned, the amount of force is all that matters. So we can keep the weight the same (our bodies) as long as we increase the amount of force we're using.

## Changing the Angle

One way to make training more difficult is simply to change the *angle* of the exercise. This is called 'extending the lever arm' which basically means that we're moving the weight (our body) further away from the point where we're applying force. This then makes the exercise more difficult because the amount of force generated has to be greater.

The easiest way to demonstrate this is by doing a press up. Get into push up position as you normally would but now, instead of performing the press up like that, you're going to move your arms *down* slightly (so that they're level with the bottoms of your pecs) and you're going to turn your hands to face slightly outward.

What you have just done is to extend the lever. You are now lifting *more weight* because your body is hanging over the top and the force needs to travel further along your arm and at an angle. Although the amount of weight hasn't changed, the amount of force *has*. This is called a

'maltese press ups' by the way.

## Increasing the Acceleration

As far as your muscle fiber is concerned, acceleration and strength are the same things. In other words, to contract your muscle *quickly* is the exact same thing as to contract your muscle *hard*.

This then means that we can now use something called 'plyometrics' in order to train the same explosive 'fast twitch' muscle fibers that we would with a heavy weight. The perfect example?

Clapping press ups! Simply perform press ups as normal but launch yourself up into the air as high as you can and clap once or twice. In doing this, you are still performing press ups with the same amount of weight but now you are launching yourself into the air through the sheer acceleration. You'll find you fatigue a lot more quickly as a result!

## How to Double the Weight

Want to quickly double the amount of weight that you're using to lift yourself during a pull up?

The very simple solution is to remove one arm from the bar. This way, you are now lifting the same amount of weight but with just one bicep, one lat and one side of your body. The same applies for press ups and tricep dips and numerous other types of exercise.

At this point you're probably wondering how you ever *get* to the point where you can perform pull ups with one hand. And the simple answer is to transition gradually! In other words, you can start by putting 70% of your weight on one hand and 30% on the other.

This requires you to manipulate the amount of force you exert on each side too and in doing that, you're improving your mind-muscle connection and also your agility and body control! Very cool.

So perform a pull up leaning slight more to one side, then move more toward the other side on the next rep and continue to alternate like that. This way, you are going to be able to gradually build up the strength to lift yourself entirely on just one side eventually!

*Using Intensity Techniques to Build Muscle With Bodyweight Moves*

As you can see then, there are plenty of ways you can make bodyweight training hard. Can you do a hand stand push up with one hand yet? Can you hold planche (arms on the maltese push up position, legs hovering behind you)? If not, then you haven't exhausted all the possibilities with bodyweight training yet!

The problem is that a lot of people just don't apply these techniques right when doing bodyweight training to try and build muscle. They do 30 press ups three times and then call it a day for pecs! Either that you they have a weak attempt at a maltese push up, or at a one handed push up and then they give up.

But remember: to accomplish the very most growth you need to increase volume and that means the amount of repetitions *and* the amount of weight.

And you need to find ways to push yourself *past* failure. If you stop before you're forced too then you won't cause those microtears and you won't trigger that much growth.

This is where we can turn to bodybuilders for inspiration. They will combine a number of different exercises in unique ways in order to push past failure and increase their volume and their time under tension. These techniques are referred to as 'intensity techniques' or the 'Joe Weider principles'.

They include things like drop sets – which involve lowering the weight each time you reach failure and then doing more reps. They also include supersets (switching quickly from one move to the next), giant sets (performing huge combinations of different exercises with no rest in between), burns (performing as much of the movement as they can once their muscles have tired out and given up), rest-pause (stopping halfway through the movement so that they aren't able to rely on momentum to help them through), pre-exhaust (exhausting one muscle group before an exercise so that the other muscles have to work on their own), cheats (cheating through the move so they can do just a couple more reps)… and more!

This is how you need to start thinking about your bodyweight training if you want to trigger maximum muscle growth.

That means that you don't just do 'three sets of ten' all the time. Instead you might use something called a 'mechanical drop set' which means that you make the weight lighter each time you fail but changing your position.
For instance, you could do:

Clapping press ups to failure ☐ Normal press ups to failure ☐ Press ups on your knees to failure

Or:

One handed pull ups to failure ☐ Two handed pull ups to failure ☐ Assisted pulls up to failure

Now you are fatiguing the fast twitch muscle fibers *multiple* times during the movement and you are pushing yourself far past failure. You've increased the weight, the time under tension and more and you should *feel* this start to burn in the muscle.

Really focus on that – listen to your body and try to feel how your muscles are responding. Can you feel the pump and the burn? Are you getting the same kind of workout from this training as you would do by lifting very heavy weights in the gym? If it doesn't feel hard enough, then you need to go back to the drawing board and start making it *harder*!

You can even use 'burns' at the end of these sequences. So once you've done as many pull ups as you can, you simply hang and perform as much of the movement as you can and *feel* the muscle burning as you do.

Who said that bodyweight workouts had to be easy?

*lit for Bodyweight Muscle Building: Push, Pull, Legs*

te that for this kind of intense training, you should avoid training the same muscle
up more than once a week. This isn't like the SSE workout because it's too much to
every body part like this every day.

stead, split your workouts into three separate days:

- ☐ Push (press ups, dips, shoulder press)

- ☐ Pull (pull ups, biceps, chin ups)

- ☐ Legs (squats, lunges, calf raises)

e multiple exercises that are similar and repeatedly push each muscle group to
lure. You can perform PPL once or twice a week and then just make sure to rest well
d eat lots of protein during your off days.

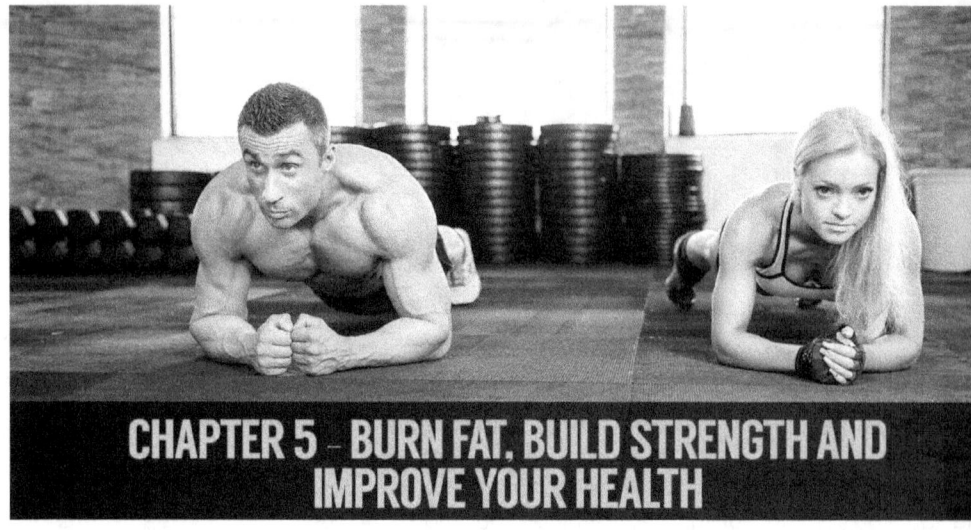

**CHAPTER 5 – BURN FAT, BUILD STRENGTH AND IMPROVE YOUR HEALTH**

## Chapter 5. Burn Fat, Build Strength and Improve Your Health

Not everyone reading this book is going to want to build big muscle though and creating intense workout splits certainly isn't for everybody.

A lot of you are going to just want to improve your health, burn some fat and feel a bit stronger. In that case, you can start seeing amazing benefits just simply by using the SSE workout we looked at at the start of this book. As you progress though, you may want to make this more challenging for yourself and spend a bit more than 10 minutes in the morning to build some real strength and burn some real fat!

### Burning Fat With Bodyweight Training

People who want to burn fat and lose weight will often mistakenly assume that they can't really achieve that using weights or bodyweight training. This is why you'll find that the majority of weight loss programs tend to revolve around cardio and aerobic exercises such as running, cycling or skipping rope.

Don't get me wrong – this *is* an effective way to burn fat.

It's just that bodyweight training is *better*. Trust me!

There are many reasons for this. The first is that bodyweight training when performed in the right way actually involves more energy than running. That's because you can use *all* of your limbs. Try performing burpees for 30 seconds and then see how you feel! It's just as energetic as running and you're burning just as many calories. And contracting at the same time only makes this even more insanely tough – this is what's known as 'resistance cardio' and it's one of the very best ways to burn fat quickly.

At the same time, performing things like burpees is *also* using a lot of muscle. You'll be using all your leg muscles, your triceps, your pecs, your shoulders... and when you do this, you trigger the release of growth hormone and testosterone. These are *anabolic* hormones that cause you to build muscle *and* burn more fat.

And what's more, is that simply *having* more muscle will also help you to burn more fat. If you have big biceps and pecs then your body needs to fuel them and that means that you'll burn through lots more calories even while you're sleeping!

There's also the fact that toning muscle at the same time as burning fat leads to a much better physique. A lot of people want to get rid of cellulite for instance. Guess what? The best way to get rid of cellulite is not to burn fat but rather to build muscle underneath and thereby tone up the flesh and make everything look smoother.

Toning muscle also gives you all the proportions you want. If you're a woman, then type in 'girls who squat' at Google Images. You'll see that women who squat are *famous* for having great buttocks. You can do the exact same thing with tuck jumps but you'll be burning more fat at the same time!

## The Workouts

So how do you put this into practice? Fortunately, it's pretty easy.

This time we *do* want to focus on whole body workouts. Doing that will enable us to burn more calories and to trigger the release of more hormones at once. And we're not going to be fatiguing the muscles to the same degree, so there's no reason we can't train the same area a few times in a row.

Circuits lend themselves perfectly to this and now all you're going to do is to make sure that you perform each 'station' with high intensity. That means that you're going to pump out as many repetitions as you can and move straight from one station to the next. Time yourself and try to beat your 'high score' each time you do the workout.

You can also throw in a few cardio moves and then just make sure that the last station gives you a decent amount of time to rest and recover before you start again.

Here's what an example might look like:

- ☐ 30 seconds pull ups

- ☐ 30 seconds clapping push ups

- ☐ 30 seconds tricep dips

- ☐ 30 seconds tuck jumps

- ☐ 30 seconds chin ups

- ☐ 30 seconds jumping lunges

- ☐ 30 seconds incline push ups

- ☐ 30 seconds rest

Then just repeat this 5 times for a 20 minute workout! You can replace the moves for things that are harder/easier depending on your ability, just make sure that you are going full throttle

(assuming you're in good health of course) and that you hit each muscle group in the body.

You can use this workout 3-5 times a week and you'll find that's more than enough to *really* start toning up.

And if you're looking for something a little more guided that will talk you through the movements, you can always try something like *The Insanity Workout*. They're actually very good.

I wouldn't though. Why? Because you can get tons of free videos on YouTube and free apps that do the *exact* same thing.

## HIIT and Tabata

Think the circuit above is too easy? Then let's up the ante a little...

HIIT stands for 'High Intensity Interval Training' and is a *very* popular form of training right now for people looking to lose weight. The basic idea of this kind of training is that you are alternating between periods of extreme exertion and gentle recovery.

So for example, you might sprint for 30 seconds and then jog for 2 minutes and repeat. This works because it allows you to switch between aerobic and anaerobic training. Aerobic training means that you are running at a speed that allows you to burn fat stores by breathing in more oxygen and circulating it. This occurs when you exert yourself at 70% of your maximum heartrate.

Conversely, anaerobic training occurs when you train at 90% of your maximum heartrate. At this point, you are exercises far too quickly in order to burn fat and so you burn sugar in the blood instead. When you do this, it means that you use up all that available sugar and from that point onward your body can *only* use fat stores. It also means that you carry on burning fat throughout the rest of the day as you have lower blood sugar.

There's more to this as well. HIIT allows you to exert yourself more in a shorter timeframe, thereby making the form of exercise much more practical and meaning that you're more likely to squeeze it into a busy schedule and get much more benefit from it.

Of course this can be applied to bodyweight training – which is already more effective than just cardio (it's 'resistance cardio') and which also triggers an anabolic response. This is the *perfect storm* for weight loss.

And it need only take you four minutes a day…

**Tabata Protocol**

The Tabata protocol is one of the best techniques available for utilizing HIIT and it takes just four minutes.

The idea is simple:

30 seconds of exercise

30 seconds of rest

And you repeat this eight times.

Sounds easy but it's absolutely brutal by the end as long as you're training with full intensity.

Good examples of things you can do include tuck jumps, press ups, pull ups (this is not easy *at all* though) or clapping push ups.

As you progress, you can also use the Tabata protocol in conjunction with 'active recovery'. That means that instead of resting for thirty seconds, you're now going to hold plank or do sit ups – some form of 'light' bodyweight training.

Don't try this until you've been doing SSE for a while or regular circuits. When you first try it, only do it for 2 minutes.

This is HARD as nails. But it really does get results.

## Training for Strength

If all you're really interested in is improving your strength, then you don't need to do Tabata and you might not want to do intense workouts that trigger maximum hypertrophy either.

In this case, what you can focus on instead is 'progressions'. This means progressing from a relatively easy exercise, all the way up to a much harder one.

You can use full body for this and you might start with a basic workout that lets you hit each body part a few times:

**Press Ups – 3 x Failure**

**Pull Ups – 3 x Failure**

**Plank – 1 Minute**

**Sit Ups – 3 x Failure**

**Decline Press Ups – 3 x Failure**

**Tuck Jumps – 3 x 1 Minute**

**Bodyweight Squats – 3 x 20**

**Calf Raises – 3 x 20**

Perform this three times a week.

en, once you start being able do these lots of times, you can begin to increase the allenge. Instead of doing press ups, you may start doing clapping press ups – or cking press ups (you'll find descriptions of these later). Likewise, you might try to ogress from decline press ups to handstand push ups with your feet against the wall.

aybe you move from plank to 'faux planche'.

en you perform this next step up until you can do all of those things very easily. And m there you make the next step up to something even harder. Now you might do anche, you might do regular handstand push ups and you might start doing clapping ess ups behind your back.

## aining for Health

nally, you can also use bodyweight training as the perfect tool for improving your erall health. In this case, you can keep your workouts fairly easy. Stick with 'full body' utines but don't worry so much about the progression. Instead, make it a part of your utine and at the same time, try to build in some light stretching and perhaps even me quiet meditation.

r overall health what's really important is just that you *move* and that you actually use ur body. Many of us aren't capable of performing a full squat movement with our els flat on the floor and this is indicative of *severe* flexibility issues. Try getting around at problem by performing body weight squats and going all the way to the ground. ewise, try to add in some cardio moves like tuck jumps to get the heart beating.

o at your own pace. At this point, you've learned *how* many of these moves are ecting your body. So all that's left to do is to find the goals you want to shoot for and gently introduce the right training into your routine.

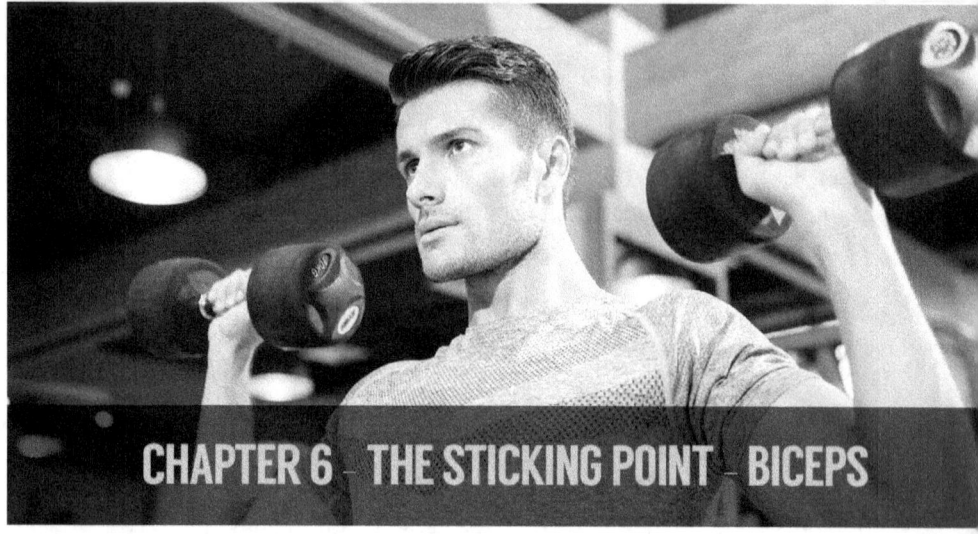

## Chapter 6. The Sticking Point – Biceps

The title of this book promises that you can get into great shape with NO equipment. And yet we *keep* mentioning pull ups and chin ups.

That's because training the biceps with zero equipment is actually quite hard. And the same is also true for the lats and pulling movements in general. A pull up bar – as we said already – can be bought online for $5 and will fit into your doorframe without even needing you to screw it in or drill any holes. There's really *no* reason that you can get one of these.

And if you can't, then there are a few more options. One is to use the underside of a table or desk. Simply lie flat underneath the table, hook your hands under one edge and then perform

'half' pull ups with your legs on the ground. Or you can even lift the legs up and do pull ups while in a 'sitting' type position.

Another option is to head outside and grab a tree branch. Or if you're the very dedicated kind, then you can grab onto the doorframe with your finger-tips. It hurts, but it works!

Option number three is to take a towel, trap it in a door (by closing it on it) and then lean backwards holding the towel and to pull yourself up that way.

There are *tons* of options in other words and I really do believe that you should be able to find *something* that works.

But if you really do want to use only your own body, there are still a couple of exercises you can use:

## Bicep Exercises With No Need for Equipment

**Elbow Curls:** This is a strange looking move but is the closest thing we have to pull ups without the pull up bar. Basically, you're going to lie on one side, with your legs bent and knees pointing in front of you. You'll also keep one arm trapped underneath those legs and under your body.

Now, using that arm, clutch onto your legs with your hand and then *pull* your body towards your legs. As you do, hinge at the elbow and raise your body off the ground.

**Curl-Grip Press:** Now you'll be in press up position but with your arms very wide apart (wider than your shoulders) and with your fingers pointing outwards. Lower yourself down slowly and as you do, you should feel the biceps contract through the 'negative' portion of the movement.

**Sitting Knee Curl:** Sit on a sofa or a chair and tuck your hands under your knees. Now you're going to curl the knees upward towards your body and you're going to use your biceps to do it.

**Ankle Curl:** Similar, is to sit on the sofa or chair and then to lift one leg up with your foot pointing at the wall on your left or right side. Take the opposite arm and grab the ankle and then curl your own foot upwards towards you in a 'concentration curl' type position. As you do this, push down against your hand with your foot and fight yourself with it.

## Dynamic Tension and Dynamic Self Resistance

There are two more methods you can use to train your biceps with your body alone. One option is to use something called 'dynamic tension'. This is the training method that was introduced by Charles Atlas and it's very simple: you just tense the biceps as hard as you can and then move through the bicep curl motion. This way, you're still contracting the muscle, you're still going through the full range of motion and you're still building the mind-muscle connection through the neuromuscular junction. In other words? It's similar to really performing a bicep curl as far as your body is concerned. Just be aware that this method won't be enough to create many microtears and as such, it's not *as* good as using actual resistance.

Another option though is 'dynamic self-resistance'. Here, you are going to curl one arm while simultaneously using your *other* arm to force it down. Perform a 'hammer curl' motion in front of your own body and just push down on your fist/forearm using the other hand. You can set the resistance yourself and this even allows you to perform a kind of 'drop set'.

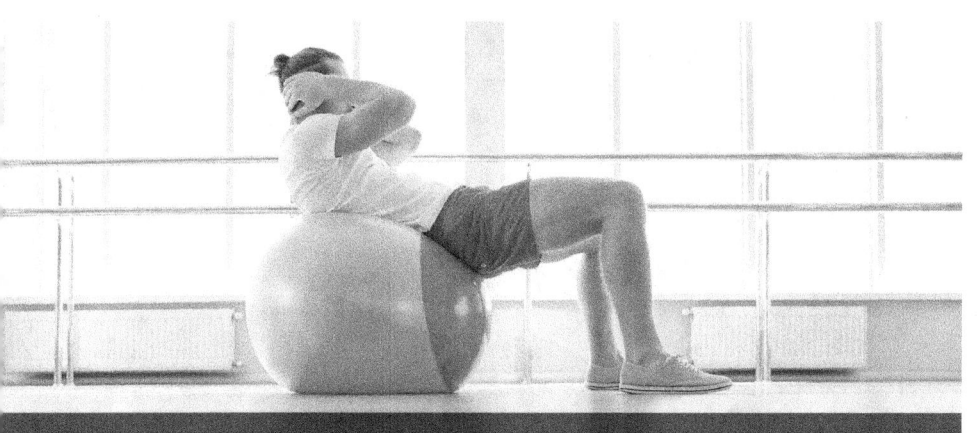

# CHAPTER 7 - A GLOSSARY OF EXERCISES

## Chapter 7. A Glossary of Exercises

Alright, now you know what you need to do and we've gotten the awkward subject of biceps out the way, it's time to look at some of the actual moves you can use!

Of course there are many more bodyweight exercises and there's nothing to stop you creating your *own* bodyweight moves either. Just use this as a starting point...

*Push Up/Dip/Handstand Variations*

**Press Ups**

You know this one! Lie flat on the ground, hands shoulder width apart and push your upper body upright.

**Clapping Push Up**

Our first variation, just perform push ups but clap in the air once.

You can also perform:

- ☐ Double claps

- ☐ Claps behind the back

## Maltese Push Up

We touched on this already: this is a push up with your hands slightly further down your body and facing outward.

## Uneven Push Ups

Push ups with one hand on a medicine ball or another raised platform.

## Wall Press Ups

For those who can't do press ups, lean against a wall and push yourself away.

## Knee Press Ups

Press ups on your knees.

## One Handed Push Ups

Like they sound. You can also do them 'Rocky style' and switch from one hand to the next mid-air.

## Incline Press Ups

Hands on something higher like a sofa. Makes it a little easier and is useful for drop sets.

## Decline Press Ups

Moves the pressure to the shoulders slightly more and the upper pecs.

## Rocking Press Ups

Push down more on one side and then more on the other.

## Diamond Press Ups

Have your fingers form a diamond shape in the middle of your chest on the ground. This is a good way to focus more on the triceps.

## Wide Grip/Narrow Grip

ves the focus to the outer pecs and the triceps respectively.

**tended Range of Motion Press Ups**

t both hands on something a little raised from the ground so you can do press ups *ther* down than you normally would.

**ps**

os can be performed on any two surfaces of the same height just opposite each other.

**icep Dips**

is is a dip but with your hands behind you on a sofa or another raised platform and et touching the ground stretched out in front.

**ke Push Up**

ish up with your body pointing down towards the ground. This works the shoulders ore once again.

**ndstand Push Ups**

th or without support!

## Supermans

Lie on the floor with your arms outstretched and then raise both your hands and feet off the ground. Hold for a second, lower and then repeat.

## Salute to the Sun

The same movement but without lifting the legs.

## Power Bridge

Lie flat on the ground with your feet on the floor and then raise your body up, propping your upper body up on your shoulders.

## Sit Ups

You know this one! Lie flat, then sit yourself up. Make sure to roll your stomach, not fold at the hips. The latter will only work your hip extensors, not your abs!

## Crunches

This is even more of a rolling motion. Your abs should 'crunch' before you make it all the way up.

## Twisting Sit Ups

Sit up and touch one elbow to the opposite knee (hands behind your head) and then repeat on the other side. Note that your hands should never 'pull' your body up, they're just there to prevent you from cheating. Twisting like this will help you to involve the obliques, which are muscles on either side of your abs.

## Leg Raises

Lie flat on the ground and raise your legs slightly to train the lower abs.

## Hanging Leg Raises

Hang from a pull up bar and then raise your legs straight up in front of you. This is similar to the 'captains chair'.

### Frog Kicks

Hang from the pull up bar then just bring your knees up to your stomach. This is an easier version of hanging leg raises and is ideal for mechanical drop sets targeting the abs!

### V Sit Ups

Lie on the ground then raise your upper body with hands outstretched to touch your toes, with legs outstretched.

### V Sits

Rest on your hands and hold your legs directly up in front of you.

### Bicycle Crunch

Like twisting sit ups except you also 'cycle' your feet as you touch your knees to your hand.

Upper body stays raised and never touches the ground.

## *Pull Up Variations*

### Pull Ups

Grab the bar with an overhand grip and pull yourself up. Arms should be fairly wide apart.

### Chin Ups

The same but with an overhand grip. This targets the biceps more.

### Around the Worlds

Use an overhand grip and move your body in a circular motion in front of the bar!

### Front Lever

An advanced move: hold the bar and then raise your legs up straight so that your body will become parallel with the ground!

**Reverse Push Ups**

Here the bar is attached closer to the ground so your legs can be outstretched and touching the floor. Take some of the weight on your heels but pull your upper body up towards the bar. (Like an 'upside down' pull up.)

**'Kipping Pull Ups'**

From CrossFit, this involves swinging your legs slightly to build momentum to get you over the bar. It allows you to perform pull ups in a more 'cardio' like manner.

**Assisted Pull Ups**

Use anything to assist you while performing pull ups. At the start of this book, we suggested using a chair!

**One Handed Pull Up**

You can also use rocking pull ups to build up to this.

**Muscle Ups**

If you have a bar with nothing above it, you can perform a pull up and go *past* the bar to then push yourself up with your pecs and shoulders.

**Neutral Grip Pull Ups**

Pull ups where you hold onto two parallel bars with palms facing inward toward each other.

**Towel Pull Ups**

Pull ups holding onto two ends of a towel draped over something. Great for building grip strength!

*Lower Body Variations*

## Bodyweight Squat

A simple squat using only bodyweight.

## Pistol Squat

A one legged squat performed with your heel on the ground and all the way to the floor. You can do a simpler one-legged squat to build up to this.

## Sissy Squat

This is a squat where you are on tip toe and you 'lean back' while bending your legs.

## Side Squat

Step out to one side and plunge deep into the movement.

## Lunge

Step forward and lunge deep on one leg with the other behind you.

## Jumping Lunges

Lunge, jump and land in the reverse lunge.

## Tuck Jumps

Jump and tuck your knees up to your chest mid-air.

## Jack-in-the-Box

Squat all the way down from a ball shape and then jump up into a starfish shape. Star jumps are an easier form of this.

## Squat Jumps

A bodyweight squat with a jump on the end.

## Calf Raises

Stand on a step or somewhere else so that your heels are hanging over the edge. Raise yourself up with just your calves.

**One Legged Calf Raises**

The same thing but with just one foot. You may need to use a free hand to suppo
yourself.


## Equipment Worth Investing In (And Getting Creative)

Want to take your training further? There is some cool equipment out there that you ca
use to make your bodyweight workouts more intense.

One great example is to get gymnastic rings. These can hang from any pull up bar an
will let you perform ring dips and even the iron cross from home!

Push up stands are also great for doing press ups through a longer range of motion.

But really, why not get a bit more creative? We've already seen that two chairs ca
make a dipping station. Three can be used to do some really deep push ups. Likewis
you can do pull ups and muscle ups from tree branches or you can hang onto a rop
and tie it around a tree.

Or how about taking cans of Coke and using them as push ups stands?

Get inventive – it's part of the fun of bodyweight training!

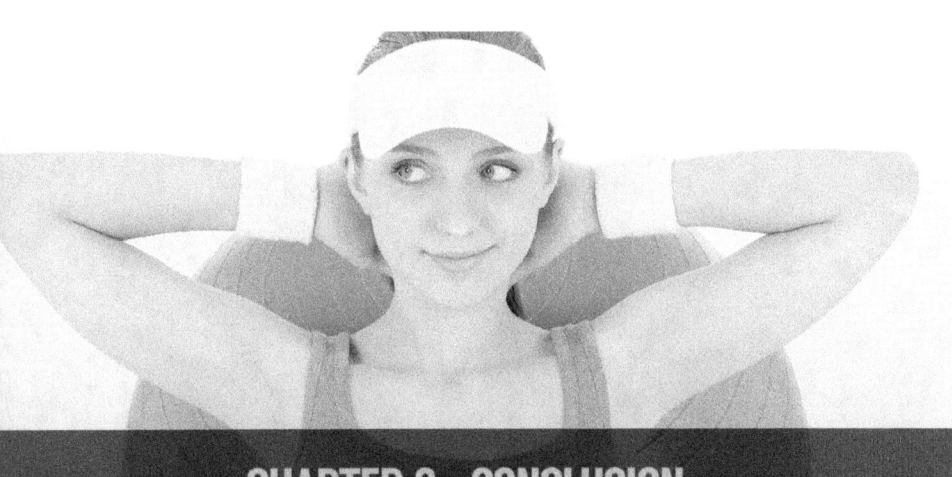

## Chapter 8. Conclusion

Combining your fast diet lifestyle with bodyweight training is desirable to burn fat, build lots of muscle and increase your overall health.

A regular workout along with your fast diet lifestyle will have number of benefits. Besides maintaining and building your muscle during fasting, it also affects your self esteem and your body image. As a whole you not only lose your weight but also feel good about yourself.

In my opinion fast diet is the best way to lose weight as well as overall improvement of your health. It is the best from the point of practicality and adaptability for a long period of time.

More than anything else it is stress free and guilt free as there is no need for you to keep on exploring new diet and weight loss plans.

Hopefully also at this point you've seen just how powerful bodyweight training can be. This is a way to work out that requires *no* equipment, that's incredibly fun and that you can do anywhere.

It can be used to burn fat, build lots of muscle and increase your overall health. And there's no reason why it can't be just as effective in building size, strength and mass as any training program in the gym. The key is to just understand how it's working and *why* it's working. Using drop sets, super sets, burns and cheats you can get just as much pump during a workout and trigger some real growth (but of course you need to eat plenty of protein to put that into action).

We've also seen how bodyweight training can be used to create *highly* intensive cardio routines and HIIT programs that will burn maximum fat and that will help you burn more calories for days afterward.

Start experimenting with these techniques and see just how much you can get out of your own bodyweight programs.

And if you're not sure where to begin? Just start doing SSE in the mornings. Those ten minutes will help you to build some initial energy, to improve your health and to add muscle. From there, you'll have a base on top of which you can begin really transforming your body with a more intensive regime.

# Quick Fast Diet Recipe Guide

**1)    Total Calories: 472**

Breakfast: Cheese & Tomato Breakfast Omelette (170 calories)

Ingredients:

- 5 sprays of rapeseed oil (22 calories)
- 35g cherry tomatoes (halved = 6 calories)
- 1/4 red onion, peeled, and finely diced (about 40g = 8 calories)
- 6 or 8 fresh basil leaves (4 calories)
- 2 small Free-Range eggs (37g each = 54 calories x 2 = 108 calories)
- 1 tablespoon grated Parmesan cheese (22 calories)
- salt and pepper

Preparation:

Heat up a small non-stick frying pan and spray the oil into it, then add the onions and fry over a gentle heat for 3 to 5 minutes or until nearly soft; add the halved cherry tomatoes and cook for a further 3 to 5 minutes or until the tomatoes are soft and just start to release their juices. Take off the heat and add the chopped basil leaves, Spoon the tomato mixture into a bowl and wipe the pan clean.

Slide the omelette out of the pan on to a warm plate and season with black pepper. Can be served as a light lunch with salad leaves, but add the calories on for that!

Dinner: Hoisin wraps (302 calories)

Ingredients:

- 200g cooked turkey or chicken, cut into strips
- 4 tbsp hoisin sauce
- 2 flour tortillas
- ¼ cucumber, deseeded and shredded
- 4 spring onions, trimmed and finely shredded
- good handful watercress

Preparation:

Heat the grill to high. Mix the turkey or chicken with half of the hoisin sauce so that it's coated, then spread out onto an ovenproof dish and grill until sizzling. Warm the tortillas under the grill or according to pack instructions.

Spread the tortillas with the rest of the hoisin sauce, then use to wrap up the turkey or chicken with the cucumber, onions and watercress. Cut in half and enjoy while still warm.

------------------------------------------------------------------------

## 2)    Total Calories: 477

Breakfast: Creamy Garlic Mushrooms on Toast, (190 calories)

Ingredients:

- Flora - Pro Active Margarine, 15 g
- Garlic Clove, 1 Medium Clove (4g) (peeled and minced)
- 100g mushrooms, wiped and peeled if necessary (cut in to slices)
- Philadelphia - Soft Cream Cheese - Full Fat - Garlic and Herb, 20 g
- Warburtons - Medium Sliced White Bread, 1 slice (23.7g)
- salt and pepper to taste
- fresh parsley (for garnish)

Preparation:

Put half the margarine into a frying pan and heat over medium heat, before adding the garlic; cook for 1 minute and then add the sliced mushrooms and cook over a low to medium heat for 5 to 7 minutes.

Meanwhile, toast the bread and spread the remaining margarine over it - cut into 4 triangles and spoon the creamy garlic mushrooms over the top, and garnish with fresh parsley.

Dinner: Sweet potato & lentil soup (287 calories)

Ingredients:

- 2 tsp medium curry powder
- 3 tbsp olive oil
- 2 onions, grated
- 1 eating apple, peeled, cored and grated
- 3 garlic cloves, crushed

- 20g pack coriander, stalks chopped
- thumb-size piece fresh root ginger, grated
- 800g sweet potatoes
- 1.2l vegetable stock

- 100g red lentils
- 300ml milk
- juice 1 lime

Preparation:

Put the curry powder into a large saucepan, then toast over a medium heat for 2 mins. Add the olive oil, stirring as the spice sizzles in the pan. Tip in the onions, apple, garlic, coriander stalks and ginger, season, then gently cook for 5 mins, stirring every so often. Meanwhile, peel, then grate the sweet potatoes. Tip into the pan with the stock, lentils, milk and seasoning, then simmer, covered, for 20 mins. Blend until smooth using a stick blender. Stir in the lime juice, check the seasoning and serve, topped with roughly-chopped coriander leaves.

-------------------------------------------------------------------------------------------

## 3)    Total Calories: 407

Breakfast: Poached egg with watercress and tomato salad (210 calories)

Ingredients:

- 2 eggs
- 1 tsp sunflower seeds
- 50g (1¾oz) watercress, roughly chopped
- 6 cherry tomatoes, finely diced
- 1 tsp finely chopped coriander

Preparation:

Bring a pan of water to the boil, take off the heat and stir the water in a circular motion for a few seconds. Crack one egg into a cup and pour into the centre of the vortex. After two minutes, shake the pan to see if the white is almost set. Remove with a slotted spoon and drain. Repeat with the other egg. Toast the seeds over a medium heat for one minute. Mix with the watercress and tomatoes. Serve the eggs on top with a sprinkle of coriander.

**Dinner: Mango Tilapia (197 calories)**

Ingredients:

- 1/4 cup canned tomato sauce
- 2 tablespoons (1 ounce) mango nectar
- 2 tablespoons ketchup
- 2 teaspoons brown sugar (loosely packed)
- 2 teaspoons cider vinegar
- 1 teaspoon molasses
- 1/2 teaspoon garlic powder
- 1/4 cup diced tomatoes
- 1/4 cup diced mango
- Two 4.5-ounce fillets raw tilapia
- 1 tablespoon chopped cilantro, for garnish

Preparation:

In a medium bowl, combine tomato sauce, mango nectar, ketchup, brown sugar, vinegar, molasses, and garlic powder. Whisk thoroughly, and then stir in diced tomatoes and mango.

Place fish and sauce in a container and toss to coat. Cover and let it marinate in the refrigerator for 30 minutes.

Bring a skillet sprayed with nonstick spray to medium heat on the stove. Add fish and marinade. Once marinade begins to simmer, cover and cook until the fish is tender and cooked through, about 5 minutes.

------------------------------------------------------------------------------------

**4)    Total Calories: 479**

Breakfast: Boiled egg with rocket and walnuts (220 calories)

Ingredients:

- 2 eggs
- 50g (1¾oz) rocket
- 2 walnuts, crushed
- ½ tsp olive oil

Preparation:

Place the eggs in boiling water for six minutes. Drain and peel. Combine the rocket, walnuts and olive oil, season and serve the eggs in quarters on top of the salad.

Dinner: Ranch Salad Recipe (259 calories)

Ingredients:

- 3/4 cup cubed cooked chicken breast
- 3/4 cup canned kidney beans, rinsed and drained
- 1 small tomato, chopped
- 1/3 cup frozen corn, thawed
- 2 tablespoons chopped red onion
- 1/4 cup ranch salad dressing
- 1 tablespoon barbecue sauce
- 1-1/2 cups torn romaine

Preparation:

In a small bowl, combine the chicken, kidney beans, tomato, corn and onion. Combine ranch dressing and barbecue sauce; pour over salad and toss to coat. Cover and refrigerate for 30 minutes. Divide romaine between two salad plates; top with salad. Yield: 2 servings.

------------------------------------------------------------------------------------------

**5)      Total Calories: 429**

Breakfast: Pumpkin & Granola Parfait (266 calories)
Ingredients:

- 1 container (6 ounces) plain low-fat yogurt
- 2teaspoons honey
- 1/4teaspoon  pumpkin-pie spice
- 1whole-grain crunchy granola bar, crumbled
- 1/2cup  canned pumpkin

Preparation:

Mix together yogurt, honey and pumpkin-pie spice. In a bowl, layer yogurt mixture, granola-bar crumbs and pumpkin.

**Dinner: Guacamole (163 calories)**

Ingredients:

- 3 avocados
- Salt
- Pico de Gallo, recipe follows
- Tortilla chips, for serving

Preparation:

Halve the avocados lengthwise. Remove the pit and dice the flesh inside the shell. Squeeze the diced avocado into a bowl.

Next, sprinkle on some salt and mash away with a fork until you get the avocado to the consistency you want.

Now throw on a big pile of Pico de Gallo and stir together gently. Always test the guacamole with tortilla chips so you'll get a more accurate gauge of the salt content.

-------------------------------------------------------------------------------------------

**6)    Total Calories: 476**

Breakfast: Spiced fruit loaf (190 calories)

Ingredients:

- 450g strong white flour, plus extra for dusting
- 2 x 7g sachets easy-blend yeast
- 50g caster sugar
- 150ml warm milk
- 1 egg, beaten
- 50g unsalted butter, melted, plus extra for greasing
- oil, for greasing
- For the spices
- 1½ tsp ground cinnamon
- 1 tsp ground ginger
- For the dried fruit
- 50g dried apricots, chopped
- 50g dried figs, chopped
- 50g pitted dates, chopped
- 50g sultanas
- 50g glacé cherries, chopped
- juice 1 orange

Preparation:

Soak the dried fruits in the orange juice for about 30 mins, then sieve, reserving the juice.

Put the flour, yeast, caster sugar and 1 tsp salt into a large mixing bowl with the spices and soaked fruit and mix well. Make a well in the centre and pour in the warm milk, reserved orange juice, the beaten egg and the melted butter. Mix everything together to form a dough – start with a wooden spoon and finish with your hands. If the dough is too dry, add a little more warm water; if it's too wet, add more flour.
Knead in the bowl or on a floured surface until the dough becomes smooth and springy. Transfer to a clean, lightly greased bowl and cover loosely with a clean, damp tea towel. Leave in a warm place to rise until roughly doubled in size – this will take about 1 hr depending on how warm the room is.

Knock the dough back by kneading for a few secs. Dust 2 x 2lb loaf tins with flour. Halve the dough. Use a little flour to help you shape each half into a smooth oval, then pop them into the tins. Cover both loosely with a clean, damp tea towel and leave to prove in a warm place for about 20 mins. Meanwhile, heat oven to 180C/160C fan/gas 4.
Bake for 20 mins, then cool in the tins before turning out and slicing.

**Dinner: Speedy meatball stew (286 calories)**

Ingredients:

- 2 medium potatoes, peeled and cut into bite-size cubes
- 1 tbsp olive oil
- 250g small lean beef meatballs
- 1 onion, chopped
- 2 garlic cloves, chopped
- 1 tbsp chopped rosemary
- 560ml jar passata
- 200g frozen peas
- few parmesan shavings, to serve (optional)

Preparation:

Boil the potatoes for 10 mins until tender. Meanwhile, heat the oil in a large saucepan. Season the meatballs, then brown them all over for about 5 mins. Remove from the pan, drain off any excess fat, then add the onion, garlic and rosemary. Fry gently for 5 mins.

Add passata to the pan, bring to a simmer, then add the meatballs. Simmer for 5 mins or until everything is cooked through. Add the potatoes and peas, then simmer for 1 min. Pack into a flask or reheat at work, add Parmesan, if using, and eat with good crusty bread.

-----------------------------------------------------------------------------------

## 7)    Total Calories: 437

Breakfast: Squash, goat's cheese & rosemary pancakes (269 calories)

Ingredients:

- 200g self-raising flour
- 1 tsp baking powder
- 1 rosemary sprig, finely chopped
- 1 egg
- 300ml milk
- 25g butter, melted and cooled, plus a knob extra
- 2 tbsp olive oil
- 250g butternut squash, peeled, deseeded and cut into small cubes
- 100g vegetarian goat's cheese, crumbled into small pieces
- handful pumpkin seeds, rocket salad and onion chutney, to serve

Preparation:

Mix the flour, baking powder, rosemary and a good pinch of salt in a large bowl. Beat the egg with the milk. Make a well in the centre of the dry ingredients and whisk in the milk mixture and melted butter to make a thick, smooth batter. Place in the fridge while you prepare the rest of the ingredients.

Over a medium heat, add a knob of butter and 1 tsp oil to a large pan, then add the butternut squash and cook for 10 mins until tender, turning the heat up for the final few mins to brown a little. Remove batter from the fridge, add the goat's cheese and squash, then carefully fold everything together.

Heat a little oil in a non-stick frying pan, then, in batches, add a ladleful of batter per pancake. Allow to cook for 3 mins until bubbles cover the surface, then flip over and cook the other side until golden. Serve with dressed rocket salad, a sprinkling of pumpkin seeds and onion chutney on the side.

Dinner: Indian chickpea & vegetable soup (168 calories)

Ingredients:

- 1 tbsp vegetable oil
- 1 large onion, chopped
- 1 tsp finely grated fresh root ginger
- 1 garlic clove, chopped
- 1 tbsp garam masala
- 850ml vegetable stock
- 2 large carrots, quartered lengthways and chopped
- 400g can chickpeas, drained
- 100g green beans, chopped

Preparation:

Heat the oil in a medium saucepan, then add the onion, ginger and garlic. Fry for 2 mins, then add the garam masala, give it 1 min more, then add the stock and carrots. Simmer for 10 mins, then add the chickpeas. Use a stick blender to whizz the soup a little. Stir in the beans and simmer for 3 mins. Pack into a flask or, if you've got a microwave at work, chill and heat up for lunch. Great with naan bread.

-------------------------------------------------------------------------------------

## 8)    Total Calories: 385

Breakfast: Yogurt with apple, blueberries and sunflower seeds (185 calories)

Ingredients:

- 150g (5½oz) plain low-fat yogurt
- ½ apple, grated
- 10 blueberries
- 10g (½oz) sunflower seeds

Preparation:
Serve the yogurt topped with fruit and seeds.

Dinner: Red lentil & sweet potato (200 calories)

Ingredients:

- 1 tbsp olive oil, plus extra for drizzling
- ½ onion, finely chopped
- 1 tsp smoked paprika, plus a little extra
- 1 small sweet potato, peeled and diced
- 140g red lentils
- 3 thyme sprigs, leaves chopped, plus a little extra to decorate (optional)
- 500ml low-sodium vegetable stock
- 1 tsp red wine vinegar
- pitta bread and vegetable sticks, to serve

Preparation:


Heat the oil in a large pan, add the onion and cook slowly until soft and golden. Tip the paprika and cook for a further 2 mins, then add the sweet potato, lentils, thyme a stock. Bring to a simmer, then cook for 20 mins or until the potato and lentils are tende Add the vinegar and some seasoning, and roughly mash the mixture until you get texture you like. Chill for 1 hr, then drizzle with olive oil, dust with the extra paprika a sprinkle with thyme sprigs, if you like. Serve with pitta bread and vegetable sticks.

# Total Bodyweight Transformation Resource Sheet

You've read the book and you know how to start transforming your body using no equipment and training anywhere that suits you.

This is the key point to take home: you don't need any equipment and there's nothing stopping you from getting the body you want right now. Don't put it off any longer!

But once you are already training and seeing those results, you may find that you wish to start pushing your training further. In that case, there are a number of cool gadgets, resources and tips you can use to get more out of your workouts. And you'll find all of that right here!

Websites

**Bodyweight Fitness Reddit**

www.reddit.com/r/bodyweightfitness

The bodyweight fitness community on Reddit does what it says on the tin. Here you'll find a highly active community of people interested in bodyweight fitness. You can check out links, ask questions, get advice and share your progress!

**Bodyspace**

http://bodyspace.bodybuilding.com/

Bodyspace is another online fitness community. This is aimed predominantly at bodybuilders, but you can find people from all walks of life here. Share your photos, comment on others and track your progress!

**Fitloop.co**

https://fitloop.co/

Looking for an alternative set of workouts you can use to start training with your own body? Fitloop.co is a great website that provides useful bodyweight programs focussing on strength. There are no tools and you can use the workouts anywhere.

**Almost Every Bodyweight Exercise Ever**

http://www.thebioneer.com/almost-every-bodyweight-exercise-ever-150-moves/

This massive list of bodyweight exercises includes 150+ moves. This is a great resource if you're looking for some new training inspiration.

## Beast Skills

http://www.beastskills.com/

If you were first attracted to bodyweight training because you wanted to be able to do cool moves like one-handed pull ups, then Beast Skills is the place you need to check out.

## Apps

http://fitness.mercola.com/sites/fitness/archive/2013/04/26/bodyweight-workout-apps.aspx

This is a list of apps that provide you with bodyweight training programs on the move!

## Tabata Protocol

http://www.tabataprotocol.com/

This website provides you with all the information you need to start using tabata.

## Equipment

One of the great things about bodyweight training is that you don't need any equipment. Nevertheless, there are some cool things that can help…

Perfect Push Ups

Use these push up stands to add a 'twist' to your push ups. Literally! This engages the shoulders and forearms more.

TRX

I'm including this on the list because you likely expect it to be here. These are straps that you can attach to your pull up bar and which will then allow you to do a range of 'suspension exercises'. They're badly over priced though, especially when compared with…

## Gymnastic Rings

Gymnastic rings cost a fraction of the price of TRX and let you do dips and things like iron cross/neutral grip pull ups on top of everything else. Ultimately, this is a much better bargain and a much better way to spend your money!

Fitness Trackers

You don't need a fitness tracker but if you're going to get one, then the best options are a Microsoft Band 2 or a top of the range FitBit. In other words, anything with a heartrate monitor which will allow you to more accurately measure your calories burned.